How to Buy High Heels

Claudia

Table of Contents

Introduction 1

1. Types of High Heels 4

2. The Best Style to Buy for Your Body Type 9

3. Things You Must Know Before Shopping for High Heels 13

4. Material and Quality Matters 17

5. Make Sure the Shoe Really Fits 23

6. Classic Pumps and Basics 27

7. Top Ten Most Expensive Brands of Heels 30

8. Buying Your High Heels Online 37

About the Author 43

Imprint 44

Introduction

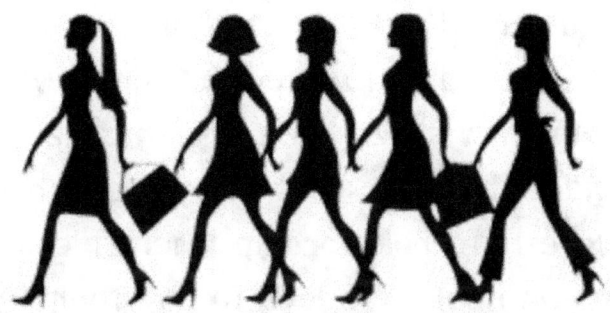

As women, what we wear is a reflection of how we feel. Our clothing choices are often based on our distinct personalities. Most of us dress according to our mood in the morning. No outfit is complete without the right accessories and that includes the shoes. We all know that the right shoes make the outfit.

Approximately 59% of women spend most of their days in high heels. We wear them to work, to go shopping, out to lunch with our friends and when we get dressed up to go out at night. When buying new shoes heels are the ones we tend to buy the most. Many of us have a love-hate relationship when it comes to high heels. We love to buy them but hate to wear them. Part of the problem is we tend to buy high heels that do not fit our feet properly.

How many times have you bought that sexy pair of heels on sale? You loved them when you bought them but ended up hating when you wore them? Sure, they felt comfortable when you tried them on in the store. But after an hour of wearing the shoes your feet were screaming at you. By the end of the day your toes were pinched or they rubbed blisters on your heels. Gone are the days when we have to sacrifice comfort for fashion. Many manufacturers have begun designing shoes that not only look great but are comfortable too. Whether you are buying heels for work or play, you can find some cute styles that you will enjoy wearing.

The tips in this guide will teach you everything you need to know to buy the perfect pair of high heels. By the time you are done reading you will know how to buy a great pair of shoes that you and your feet will love. You will learn the right shoes to buy for your body type. What you should look for before making a purchase. And most of all, the proper way to buy heels that fit your feet.

1. Types of High Heels

So many heels, so many choices. Gone are the days when high heels only came in three basic styles; pumps, mules and slings. Fashion has become fun and downright funky. Today, you can find any style shoe to fit your mood. Heels come in more heights and styles than ever before. Low heels are more suitable for work or casual outings. Mid heels offer all of the sex appeal of the high heels but are more comfortable to wear. And high heels are now even higher. Knowing what types of high heels work best for you will make it easier to buy the perfect pair.

Kitten heels were introduced back in the 1950's. The shoes are just as adorable as the name. Kitten heels have a stiletto style heel but are only about

1 to 1 ½ inches tall. You can find them in open toed, sandal and pump styles. These shoes are the perfect heel for long days on your feet when you need to look fabulous.

Pumps are the classic heel style. Every woman should own a good pair of pumps in basic black. Most pumps are two to three inches high. Pumps are generally wider than most heels and this helps to make the pointed toe more comfortable.

Platform heels are very trendy now. These heels can be either low or high, or anywhere in between. Platforms have a thicker base under the sole. Many women prefer a platform to a traditional high heel because the height difference between the front of the shoe and the back is not as steep.

Ankle-strap heels are another style that comes with all heel heights. The shoes have a supporting strap around the ankle. This detail not only makes them look sexier it acts to make them easier to walk in.

Stilettos are the highest of the high heels. The heel can range from 3 inches up to 8 inches. Walking in these stylish shoes does take some practice. If you can manage to walk gracefully in stilettos you will be sure to attract attention.

Wedge heels give you style and comfort in one great shoe. The heels have the height of pumps or stilettos but the soles are solid. These shoes are much easier to walk in than most heels and are the most comfortable to wear.

Cone heels are wider at the base. The heel becomes quite narrow at the bottom, like a stiletto. The styles of shoes with cone heels vary from sandals, to pumps to ankle straps and the heels can be low to high.

Sling backs are similar to the ankle strap heels. Instead of the strap going around the ankle, it runs around the back of the heel. This makes the heel more stable while adding a touch of elegance to the shoe.

Mules are any type of high heel that covers a large portion of the foot. The height of the heel will vary depending on the style of the shoe. Most mules just slip right onto the foot without any type of supporting strap. They may come in closed toe or peep toe styles.

Peep toe heels are defined as any shoe that shows a bit of toe. You will mainly find these in pump styles. Many women prefer the peep toe to the classic pump as they do not pinch their toes together. Peep toe heels look best when your toenails are nicely polished.

Chunky heels go in and out of fashion depending on current designer trends. The wide, square heel gives you more support when walking. These heels comes in all heights and are usually made from wood or cork. The cork soles provide added comfort due to their spongy nature.

2. The Best Style to Buy for Your Body Type

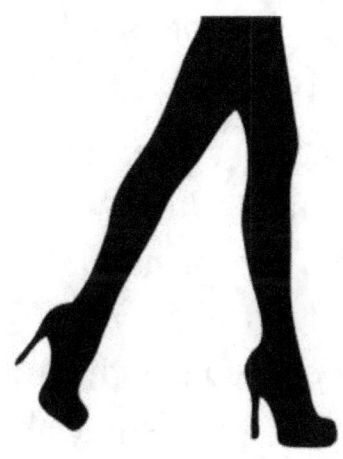

Most women know how to buy clothes to fit their body type. Vertical stripes are good for short women or ones with a fuller figure because they create a longer, leaner look. We all know that black is slimming and horizontal stripes should not be worn by most of us. But did you know that you should also buy your heels according to body type?

Short women should avoid certain styles of high heels as they can make them appear even shorter. Knowing what your body type is will help you to buy the perfect shoe.

If you have **short legs**, and want them to appear longer, stay away from ankle straps. The straps around the ankles can actually make your legs look shorter by cutting off the leg from the foot. To make your legs look longer go for sling backs or pumps. To give you added length buy heels that are at least two to three inches high. Peep toe shoes also give the impression of added length.

Women with wide feet should avoid pumps or even peep toe styles. These shoes get narrower at the toes. You should also stay away from sandal styles with lots of straps. The best choices for wide feet are mules, wedges or chunky heels. The wider heels will give you more support. Also look for heels with a rounded or open toe as they will be more comfortable.

If you have **thick ankles** do not buy the stylish stilettos or platforms. You need more support in order to look graceful in your heels while walking or dancing. Go for styles with a wedge, cork or chunky heel. Stay away from ankle straps as they tend to focus attention to the problem area. Instead go for a peep toe style that draws attention to your pretty toes. Wedge style heels are the best choice as they tend to balance out the look of thick ankles and calves.

Petite women should not buy platforms or chunky heels. The larger heels are not appealing on your smaller frame.

The perfect shoes for you are stilettos or the shorter kitten heels. These will give you the appearance of height without detracting from your smaller size.

3. Things You Must Know Before Shopping for High Heels

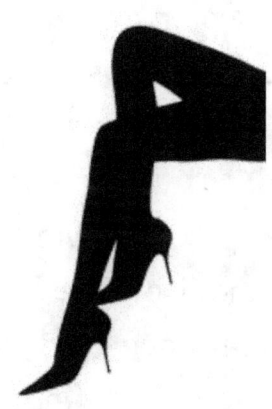

Before running out and spending your hard earned cash on those sexy pair of heels, there are a few things you should know. First determine what you are buying them for. Are the shoes for work or going out? If you are buying them for work, do you sit at a desk most of the day or are you on your feet? If the shoes are for a special event or occasion, is the event indoors or outdoors?

We have already covered how to buy the perfect pair of heels based on your body type. Now it is time to talk about the right shoes for the right occasion. You would not wear the sexy stiletto heels to a job interview or to work if you spend most of the day on your feet. Stiletto heels are also not practical if the event you are going to is outdoors. You don't want to get stuck in the grass or dirt with every step you take.

First decide what you are buying the shoes for. For work always opt for a classic look like a pump, peep toe or mule. Be sure to go with a low to mid heel so that your feet will last throughout the day. There is nothing worse than having your feet screaming at you midway through the workday because you wore the wrong shoes.

Save the sexy, strappy sandals or stilettos for a night out. Again be sure to buy the right style for your body type so your feet don't quit before the night is through. If you are going to be dancing the night away make sure the heel is appropriate for that, like a cute platform or chunky style.

All humans are not created equal. When it comes to body parts that come in pairs, like our eyes, one is always slightly larger than the other. This is true for feet too. Make sure you have your feet measured before even trying on any shoe. The shoe section in a department store is the best place to have this done. Get one of the sales people to help you so that you know exactly what size both of your feet are. Make sure that you are standing up for this. Your feet flatten and become wider when you are in a standing position.

You should always go shopping for shoes at the end of your day. Believe it or not, the size of your feet change throughout the day. Shoes that feel comfortable in the morning can often cause discomfort by the afternoon. Your feet swell during the day, so to get the best fit, shop for shoes in the late afternoon to early evening.

4. Material and Quality Matters

Ever bought a fabulous pair of shoes on sale just to have them fall apart after a few days? I am sure the answer to that question is yes, as this has happened to most of us. The old saying "you get what you pay for" holds true when it comes to buying good quality shoes. Getting a cute pair of heels on sale is great. But there are a few things you should look for before making that purchase. You want to make sure that you will get your money's worth from the shoes or you haven't really saved anything.

One of the first things to look at is **the sole**, or bottom, of the shoe. Soles are either stitched or glued on. If the sole is stitched check to make sure that the stitches are evenly spaced and sewn securely. For glued on soles, make sure there is not any part of the sole that is separated from the shoe. Poorly made shoes often have soles that are not properly attached and fall off quickly.

Check **the bottom of the heel** for an attachment to prevent slipping. Most of these will be made of rubber. Heels without this attachment can be dangerous to wear. Looking graceful is difficult if you are slipping and falling everywhere.

Make sure you look at **the lining of the shoe**. What material is used and does it completely cover the inside of the heel? Look for leather lining, it molds to the foot and absorbs moisture. Synthetic lining does not allow the foot to breath and will cause sweating. Be sure the lining completely covers the inside. Lining on only the bottom of the shoe may cause friction on the sides of your feet resulting in blisters.

When checking the lining of the shoe look for **cushioned insoles**. You want to have a cushion in the three main areas of your foot; heel, arch and the ball (just behind the toes). No cushioning means there is nothing to absorb the shock to the bones of the foot. You need this padding to keep your feet comfortable and prevent the buildup of callouses.

Material matters so buy shoes made of the finest material. **Leather** is the best choice as it conforms to the foot. Your leather heels will last longer and be the most comfortable to wear. For those folks who are against wearing any products made by animals you can find some great options in vegan leather.

Try to **avoid synthetic material or plastic**. You will not get as much wear from the shoes nor will they be as comfortable as leather. Synthetic material is not designed to allow air in. This often cause the foot to sweat and your feet will be slipping and sliding around inside the shoe. This slipping leads to friction which in turn leads to sore, blistered toes and feet.

Pay attention to the **color and style** of the shoes. Will this pair of shoes go with most of the clothes in your wardrobe? Is the style one that will quickly be outdated? Even if you buy the shoes on sale you will not save much if they end up sitting in your closet because you have nothing to go with them.

Buy shoes that go with everything. You can't go wrong with **a classic pair of black pumps**. You can dress them down for daytime or dress them up for a night on the town. These shoes never go out of style and if made from high quality material will last through several seasons of wear.

When buying colored shoes stick with a **solid color**. Sure, the animal prints or metallic may be fun now, but will they be in style in a few months? If you are looking for just the right shoes to go with a particular outfit, wear the outfit or take it with you. This way you can avoid the hassle of having to return them later when you realize they are not the shade you wanted. Many department stores offer to dye a basic pair of white shoes to match the color that you need.

You can save a lot of time, and money, by investing in one or two pairs of good quality heels. Keep the style simple and in a basic color and they will go with most everything you wear. Stick with a classic pump, peep toe or sling back in black and white. You will get more wear out of a good quality pair of heels than multiple pairs bought on sale.

5. Make Sure the Shoe Really Fits

Healthy feet are happy feet. Wearing shoes that do not fit properly can lead to many foot related health issues. Painful blisters, corns, bunions and callouses are just a few of these. The best way to avoid any of these is to buy the proper shoes. For a good fit look for a **material that conforms to your foot**, like leather. The upper part of the shoe should be sturdy enough to support your foot but give with your foot when walking. You want your feet to be able to breathe while in the shoe. Avoid shoes that cause your foot to slip and slide on the inside while wearing them. Shoes that fit too tightly will also cause friction to occur which leads to callouses and blisters forming.

Use the same **thumb rule** for buying high heels that you use for sneakers and boots. There should be a thumb space from the inside front of the shoe to your longest toe. Make sure to check this while you are standing up, not sitting down. Be sure that you have some space between your toes and the material on top of the shoe. Again, while standing, wiggle your toes in the shoes to check for this.

Open toed shoes will give your toes more wiggle room. This can be especially important for women with wide feet. Go for a sexy, black pump with a peep toe. This style of shoe never goes out of style and looks great with everything from jeans to dresses.

When buying clothes have you ever noticed that a size six is not the same size according to designers? One brand of jeans in a size six may be too small, while another fits just right. This same rule applies to the different brands of shoes. While you may be a size six according to Gucci, you will likely need a six and half in Christian Louboutin's. Don't be afraid to buy a size large if it fits better.

When trying on shoes, **walk around**. Don't just take a couple of practice steps in them. Many women do not know that most shoe departments add an extra layer of padding to their carpets. While the shoes may feel comfortable while in that department they may not be comfortable elsewhere. If you can walk into another area of the store, do so. Try to find an area with hard flooring, like tile, to check the comfort level of the heel before buying it.

Don't buy the stilettos if you are not able to walk in them. The shoes may look sexy but not if you are stumbling around while wearing them. And a swollen, sprained ankle is also not attractive. Buy a heel height you are comfortable with. Two to three inches is perfect for the work place or job interview. If you will be on your feet all day stick with one and half to two inch heels. For that special night out, three to five inches may work if you can walk in them comfortably.

6. Classic Pumps and Basics

We have already determined that every woman should have a pair of **classic black pumps** in her closet. But most of us like a little variety in our lives, and our closets. The following are some of the basics that should also be included in your wardrobe. You can use this handy list when spring cleaning your closet or before shopping for a new pair of high heels.

A stylish **pair of wedges**. You need to have at least one pair of these for your more casual looks. Wedges will give you the height you need while still being comfortable to wear. You can pair them with jeans, a sundress and even shorts in the summertime.

High heeled ankle boots are always in style. These boots are perfect for fall and winter and work wonderfully for full figured women. You can get the look of boots with your favorite jeans without the hassle of finding tall boots to fit both your feet and calves.

Full length boots are one of the top fashion accessories you need for the colder months. Go with a mid to high heel for the office and a platform or stiletto style for going out. Boots paired with jeans and a sweater never go out of style. You can also pair them with a longer skirt and blazer for the office. To dress them up go with a higher heel and shorter hem line, like a min dress and great pair of knee high boots.

Strappy sandals are another basic that should be in your closet. You can buy these in fun, flirty styles to go with your summer basics, like sundresses and shorts. Or you can buy them in barely there styles for an elegant look to wear out on the town. A sexy pair of metallic strappy heels work to dress up any outfit, but may not be appropriate in the work place.

Even if you are a lover of the very high heels, you should invest in at least **one pair of low heels**. Giving your feet a break from the constant pressure of high heels is important. A nice pair of one to one and half inch heels will still give you some of the height you want. You should wear a shorter heel on days when you will be doing a lot of walking, like shopping.

7. Top Ten Most Expensive Brands of Heels

If you are a fan of any of the reality "housewives" shows, you have probably seen their expensive shoes. Most celebrities spend more on shoes than you can make working full time in a year. And just think, some of these ladies have hundreds of pairs of them lined up in their closets. Here is a look at the top ten most expensive shoe manufacturers and where you can go to buy them, if you are lucky enough to afford them.

One of the most known, and respected, names in fashion would have to be **Gucci**. The designer from Florence, Italy is not only known for fashionable heels but they are considered by many to be the most comfortable. You can find them in their store on Rodeo Drive in Hollywood and at most of the high end department stores, like Nordstroms. A basic pair of high heels from Gucci starts around $600 and goes upwards from there.

If you are looking for fresh and trendy you need to check out **Mui Mui**. The granddaughter of Mario Prada specializes in ankle boots with stiletto heels in an eclectic mix of materials. The price range starts around $500 and goes from there. If you happen to be on Rodeo Drive they are located just three doors down from the Gucci store.

Still shopping on Rodeo Drive, about a block up the street from Gucci, you will find **Stuart Weitzman**. Although this company originally started in the United States all of his shoes are now manufactured in Spain. Stuart Weitzman combines unusual materials, like cork and 24k gold, to give a new spin on classic peep toes and pumps. Once a year he designs a pair of heels for one of the Oscar nominees that is rumored to be worth one million dollars. The starting price for a basic pair of his shoes is around $600.

Next on the list of the most expensive heels is **Brian Atwood**. You will not find him on Rodeo Drive but rather in New York on Madison Avenue. Like most designer shoes he has a manufacturing plant in Italy and is most known for his thigh high boots. A basic pair of Brian Atwood shoes starts around $600 while his boots start at $2,000.

If you are looking for something one-of-a-kind, in the fantasy heel category, you need a pair of **Alexander**

McQueen's. This former costume designer, turned shoe manufacturer, combines old world design with distinct flourishes and new age styles to create fantasy high heels. The average price for a pair of his shoes will set you back about $1500.

Walter Steiger shoes are highly sought after. He likes to combine curvy heels with fresh materials and innovative designs. While his most basic pair of shoes start around the $500 mark most of them sell somewhere in the thousands.

When talking about high end designers **Christian Louboutin** is sure to be mentioned. His shoes are best known for their red soles and very high heels. He has a whole group of people in his company whose only job is to find places to buy the red soles, that is how popular they have become. You can find his iconic shoes at Barney's New York where the most expensive pair to date was a mere $3,095.

One of the most popular high heel designers worn by the Hollywood elite are **Jimmy Choo**. You will find more than one pair on any red carpet event. His shoes were made popular in the 1980's and are known for their fun, colorful designs. One pair of these stylish heels will run you a couple thousand dollars.

Manolo Blahnik pumps came out in the 1970's during the age of high heeled boots and platform shoes. Carrie from Sex in the City was one of the reasons they are now so popular. These designer shoes can be recognized by their high stiletto heels and exotic materials, like alligator, that they are made from. You can find Manolo Blahnik's at Barneys New York where the average price is around $3,500.

And you cannot talk high end designers without **Louis Vuitton** making the list. The company has been making trendy, designer purses, luggage and shoes for the elite of society since 1854. The most expensive shoes by Louis Vuitton are not high heels but surprisingly one of their men's shoes which, at $10,000 a pair, makes them the most expensive shoes in the world.

Are these expensive designers really worth the money they cost? That depends on what you are looking for. One of the biggest differences between heels made from name brand designers and the ones you find at say, Wal-Mart, is the attention to detail. Name brand designers will only use the best quality material, for example a leather sole and not just a leather upper. While their prices are higher their shoes will wear longer.

Another difference is in the way the shoes fit. Name brand designers do not make shoes for the average woman. Your cheaper designers make shoes to fit everyone while the more expensive ones will fit a few. They also have more padding to absorb the shock to the foot than the cheaper ones. If you can afford a more expensive high heel it would be best to go with one that is classic in design so that you will get more wear from them.

8. Buying Your High Heels Online

You can find some great deals on high heels online. Before making that online purchase follow the tips outlined in this guide in a retail outlet first. Know the exact size of both of your feet and try on shoes by a variety of designers. Remember to look at comfort and fit before the actual size. Doing this before any online purchase will help you to buy a pair of heels that you are happy with and that fit you properly.

Buying shoes online has both advantages and disadvantages. One of the advantages is that you can shop in your pajamas. You can also save time by comparing prices without having to go to the mall. With just a couple of clicks of the mouse, you can see all of the latest styles at one time.

The biggest disadvantage to buying your high heels online is you cannot try them on before you buy them. Just because they look good on the website does not mean they will look good on your feet. When buying designer heels online, check to make sure they are coming directly from the designer. You do not want to waste your hard earned dollars on knock offs. Be sure to read the return policy before making any online purchase.

To help you get started shopping online here are some of the top sites in both the United States and the United Kingdom to buy high heels.

Most everyone woman has seen the commercials for **Just Fab**. The company works similar to a book club.

When you join as a member they will have you take a quick shoe survey. Once you complete the survey they will show you a selection of shoes based on your answers. The first order is buy one pair get one free and they offer free shipping. One of the drawbacks is they have a limited number of sizes available.

Heels.com has over 140 brands from you to choose from. When you subscribe to their newsletter they will send you a 10% off code towards your first purchase. They also offer free shipping and free returns. The price range here is from about $50 up to a couple of hundred depending on the style of the shoe and name brand.

Designer Shoe Warehouse is another of the big ones. They have both online and retail stores available. They have thousands of shoes to select from. DSW offers free shipping and free exchanges. One of the perks here is that you can exchange shoes bought online at any of their physical store locations.

Zappos not only offers some great deals on high heels but has clothing and home products too. While the range of styles may not be as great as some of the other sites, their price range is affordable for most. One of the interesting things with this company is that they offer free returns for one year, instead of the usual thirty days. You will also get free shipping on any order.

Number five on the US list is **Shoes.com**. The site offers over 250 brands to choose from but you will not find the bigger brand names here. The average price range is from $39.95 to around $200. Shoes.com does give you the standard free shipping but you will pay the shipping costs on any returns.

All of these sites use the standard payment methods of Visa, Mastercard and American Express credit and debit cards. Zappos has their own Visa rewards card that you can apply for. You can earn points and for every 2,500 points earned they send you a $25 gift certificate to spend with them.

For an affordable selection of sky high heels in the **Uk** check out **Quiz Clothing**. They offer a wide variety of the latest styles and brand names. They have a couple of different delivery options for you to choose from. For orders placed online to be picked up in one of their retail locations there is no charge. And for orders over sixty pounds the delivery is free.

Zalando offers heels of every height and style. The prices are geared towards the average woman. They offer free shipping and returns with a one hundred day return policy. Unfortunately they only carry shoes in whole sizes so if you are one of the many women who wears a 6 $\frac{1}{2}$ this is not the site for you.

About the Author

Claudia is the pen name of a fashion journalist of Belgian origin. She is the daughter of a banker-married couple and has lived many years in Paris, where she became familiar with the French haute couture. She is married and lives near Munich.

Imprint

www.ingramcontent.com/pod-product-compliance
Lightning Source LLC
Chambersburg PA
CBHW071257280526
45788CB00004B/1751